HEALING WITH PALEO

A STEP BY STEP GUIDE TO THE PALEO AUTOIMMUNE PROTOCOL

To: Susan

Best in health,

Dr. Jamie Koonce

DrJamieKoonce.com

BY: JAMIE KOONCE, MS, L.AC

www.Energized.Life

D1533956

Publishing services provided by 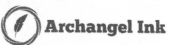 Archangel Ink

ISBN: 151731383X
ISBN-13: 978-1517313838

Table of Contents

Introduction: Why I Wrote This Book

If you picked up this book, you've probably already read about the Paleo Autoimmune Protocol on various blogs or heard about it from a friend. Perhaps you've read other books that tell you the whys and the hows of the autoimmune protocol, but you've been left feeling a bit confused. This book is less about the "whys" of the Paleo Autoimmune Protocol (or the paleo diet in general), and more about the "how to" for real people who want to do the Paleo Autoimmune Protocol without having to learn how to make the perfect autoimmune protocol donut or an enticing autoimmune protocol cricket paella.

Let's face it. If you're sick with an autoimmune condition such as Hashimoto's, celiac, rheumatoid arthritis, multiple sclerosis, Crohn's, ulcerative colitis, alopecia, chronic fatigue, fibromyalgia, lupus, Graves' disease, type 1 diabetes, lichen planus, ankylosing spondylitis, or one of the many other autoimmune conditions out there, you simply don't have the energy to sift through piles of information just to try to figure out what's "safe" to eat.

You could literally spend years reading every blog post of every blogger on the Paleo Autoimmune Protocol, and several more years reading all the books. And you know what you would find? Contradictions everywhere! One blog or podcast says you should eat plenty of carbohydrates in the form of sweet potatoes and plantains, while another paleo expert says you should eat a low-carbohydrate, high-fat, ketogenic paleo autoimmune diet. And on top of that, there are acronyms such as FODMAPs, SCD, GAPS, SIBO, and DDP that are enough to make your head spin. (Just kidding about the acronym DDP. So far, there's no one blogging about the DDP diet.) I'll address some of these contradictions and acronyms later in this book.

So let's get back to the Paleo Autoimmune Protocol thingy. There's too much info in the blogosphere if you're trying to heal, and you simply don't have time to read through it all. And it's confusing. As a Functional Medicine Practitioner and Licensed Acupuncturist, I get tons of questions from patients. And I know what you're thinking:

Does wheatgrass contain gluten? Is buckwheat a kind of wheat? Do I really have to eat cricket protein? What can I eat for breakfast if I can't have grains, eggs, dairy, nuts, or seeds? And what do I drink in the mornings if I can't have my coffee?! And now I read that I can't even have chocolate on this diet. Does anyone actually do the Paleo Autoimmune Protocol? Is it going to work? Remind me why all these foods are bad if I have an autoimmune disease!

The purpose of this book is to answer these questions and make the Paleo Autoimmune Protocol less complicated than it seems. After all, no special diet is going to work if it makes you crazy trying to figure out what to eat and what to avoid.

Also remember this: In the 1940s, the German physician Marcus Herz reportedly said, "My dear friend, an error of the press will assuredly, some day or other, be the death of you." He was referring to illegible handwriting of physicians writing prescriptions for medications. The quote eventually evolved to "Be careful reading health books. You may die of a misprint." There are still so many things that we don't understand about nutrition, so please don't let anything you read overpower your body's natural wisdom. I believe that your health will improve if you take action on the information in this book and start putting it into practice right away, but please don't take it all too seriously. There is no perfect diet for every body at every stage of life. What worked for you five years ago may not be working for you now, and what works for you now may not be what works for you in five years. Having good health is a constant process of checking in with your own body.

Why Bother with This Dietary Protocol?

Why would you put yourself through the hassles of the Paleo Autoimmune Protocol in the first place? Besides the fact that everyone online seems to be doing it and putting their autoimmune condition into remission (and telling the world about it through their blog, recipe book, Instagram feed, Facebook, Twitter, etc.), the reason behind all this madness is actually very simple. You don't have to be a scientist with a PhD to understand the whys. You don't need to pore over ten-foot-tall stacks of scholarly journals to understand why beans and grains and nuts and dairy and nightshades and other things are your kryptonite.

The bare bones of it all is this: For centuries, medical scholars and doctors in every culture on Earth believed that the root cause of most chronic illness actually lies in the gut. I learned this central theme in Chinese medical school. A doctor named Li Dong-Yuan wrote a book called *The Pi-Wei Lun* (translated to English as *The Treatise on the Spleen & Stomach*) centuries ago, and it has become one of the most important textbooks used in modern Chinese Medicine. The basic gist of the book is that many of the "complex" diseases have a root cause of immunodeficiency and digestive dysfunction. Modern science has now "discovered" that 80% of our immune system is located in the gut, but the ancient Chinese already knew this. Doctors in ancient Europe also knew that the gut was involved in chronic disease. Remember studying about Hippocrates and one of his most famous quotes? "Let food be thy medicine and medicine be thy food."

How We Forgot That Death Begins in the Colon

So this idea that the health of your digestive tract (primarily your intestines) and your immune system are intertwined, and the idea that dysfunction in these systems of the body are related to chronic disease—primarily autoimmune disease—is nothing new. But this information was forgotten—or suppressed—sometime around the late 1800s. Any talk about having a healthy gut to prevent or reverse chronic disease was passed off as an "old wives' tale" or pure quackery.

So what changed? Well, in the old days, basic information about the proper care of the human body was passed down through family lineages. Not everyone agreed 100% on everything. Doctors were free to practice any kind of therapies they found to be effective clinically. There were homeopaths, herbalists, acupuncturists, bonesetters (chiropractors), yoga instructors, and more. If you had something wrong with your health, you could go to a physician of your choosing. Of course, that physician may have given you a pill containing mercury, or they may have done some bloodletting. It was a free market. If the village healer was known for killing their patients, they weren't the village healer for very long. The free market decided who was a good doctor and who was a charlatan.

As germ theory began to catch on during the 1800s, there were some serious debates about how disease spreads. Some believed disease was airborne and that "bad air" could literally wipe out a city. Others believed disease was spread through physical contact only. As we now know, both theories are correct depending on the disease in question. We also know now that disease can spread through social networks—even online social networks. For instance, if the people in your social circle start gaining weight because they are too busy to cook for themselves, get adequate amounts of rest, and exercise, then you are more likely to gain weight as well. On the other hand, if your friends are all posting photos of their homemade "real food" lunch packed in a stainless steel lunch box, and they're going to yoga class several days a week, then you're more likely to give in to the "peer pressure" and do the same. But I digress.

The various types of healers in the 1800s couldn't agree on how disease spread throughout the population, and they couldn't agree on the appropriate method of treatment. Some said if you have a fever and sore throat, you should get plenty of rest and eat hot chicken soup. Others said you needed bloodletting to let out the excess heat. And still others thought you needed a pill.

To solve this disagreement and to protect the public from going to a charlatan doctor, the American Medical Association was founded. Only doctors who had gone to universities approved by the American Medical Association were allowed to call themselves doctors. This meant the homeopaths, naturopaths, herbalists, acupuncturists, bonesetters, and others could no longer practice medicine or refer to themselves as doctors.

Traditional wisdom about the proper care of the human body was tossed aside. The medical schools with American Medical Association approval only taught the knowledge that was new and in fashion at the time: the germ theory of disease. In 1897, the French physician Ernest Duchesne used the mold *Penicillium glaucum* to cure guinea pigs infected with typhoid. Then thirty-one years later, in 1927, Alexander Fleming accidentally discovered that *Penicillium rubens* repressed the growth of *Staphylococcus* bacteria in a petri dish. This was the beginning of antibiotic therapy as we know it today. It took two decades for antibiotics to be mass-produced by the pharmaceutical industry, and there's no doubt that the germ theory of disease and antibiotic therapy has saved countless lives.

However, with all of this scientific advancement and regulation of knowledge taught in the medical schools, there was a lack of focus on what causes chronic disease. The idea that the health of the body as a whole is closely related to the health of the gut was not something that was even considered. Scientists were learning how to isolate particular compounds from whole plant ingredients and then patent them as medicines. The "real" doctors were taught how to use these medicines to cure disease. Medications such as morphine, heroin, and cocaine—owned by Merck and Bayer—were important pain relievers during the early 1900s. There was little scientific interest in the root cause of chronic pain because these medications were widely available.

But history tends to repeat itself. Now modern scientists are finding that the health of the gut is just as important as it was believed to be back during the days of Hippocrates and Li Dong-Yuan. Just as antibiotics weren't really used in mainstream medicine until the 1940s (over four decades after penicillin was found to cure typhoid), it will probably be several years before the idea of healing the gut to reverse chronic disease enters mainstream medicine. So don't expect your conventionally trained medical doctor to mention that healing your gut might actually help you control the symptoms of your autoimmune disease or even reverse the autoimmune process. However, scientists do now know that there's a new epidemic on the rise—and it starts in the gut.

The Gut-Immune Connection

Y ou may have heard of "leaky gut," and you're probably wondering if it's real. Your doctor may say it's hogwash. The actual medical term for the condition is intestinal hyperpermeability or increased intestinal permeability. In order to understand what this is, you have to understand what happens in a healthy gut. You absorb nutrients from your food through your intestinal lining into your bloodstream. In order for this to happen, your gut has to be semi-permeable. When your food has been efficiently digested, the nutrients needed by your body are absorbed through your gut. Irritation to the gut lining can cause your gut to become too permeable. This means you start absorbing things into your bloodstream before they are completely digested. You will even absorb nasty toxins such as bacterial antigens and metabolic wastes into your bloodstream. Then your body stages an attack against these incompletely digested foreign substances. The end result is an attack against your own body's tissues—otherwise known as autoimmunity.

The increased gut permeability causes a vicious cycle to occur. You begin to develop new food sensitivities and allergies because your leaky gut is allowing food particles to be absorbed before they are completely broken down by the digestive process. Then you aren't able to get adequate nutrition, no matter how nutrient-dense your diet is. You get weaker and weaker as your body becomes more and more deficient in important micronutrients.

The theory behind the Paleo Autoimmune Protocol is that it eliminates the major food groups that can cause irritation to the gut. (I think it's actually much more complicated than that, which I'll explain later in this book.) The purpose is to stop the vicious cycle of gut hyperpermeability, your body's attack against undigested food particles entering your bloodstream, and autoimmunity. You won't have to do the Paleo Autoimmune Protocol for life. The key is to do it long enough to allow your gut to heal. Basically, you are supposed to continue the Paleo Autoimmune Protocol until your gut regains the semi-permeability that prevents undigested food particles from "leaking" into your bloodstream.

How long does it take to heal a leaky gut? And how do you know that you've regained the integrity of your gut? Some say you should introduce a non-Paleo Autoimmune Protocol food (such as eggs or nuts) one at a time and wait to see if you have a bad reaction to it. This is one way you could do it, but I don't recommend it. What if your symptoms are severe? It's too much of a gamble. The best way of starting the Paleo Autoimmune Protocol, as well as stopping it, is to test. The principle of the thing is to heal your gut, so you want to verify that you actually have leaky gut in the first place.

If you have been diagnosed with an autoimmune condition, I can guarantee you that you have a leaky gut. Li Dong-Yuan knew it, Hippocrates knew it, and now modern scientists who study the relationship between autoimmune disease and gut health know it. Before embarking on a major dietary change in an effort to heal your leaky gut, you should get a baseline of how permeable your gut is. This way you can test for improvement in your gut integrity before you start adding new foods in. By testing instead of guessing, you won't have to risk having a major setback in your healing process by introducing a new food too soon.

The traditional test for intestinal permeability requires a urine sample. To do the test, you will drink a "challenge drink" containing lactulose and mannitol (two non-metabolized sugar molecules). You will then collect your urine over the next six hours. Finally, you'll send your sample to a specialized functional medicine lab. The lab will then look at the amount of lactulose and mannitol in your urine, as well as the lactulose/mannitol ratio. An elevated lactulose/mannitol ratio or a normal lactulose/mannitol ratio with a depressed amount of mannitol is indicative of increased intestinal permeability (leaky gut).

A newer test for intestinal permeability, available only through Cyrex Labs, requires a blood serum sample. Your blood is then screened for actomyosin IgA, occludin/zonulin IgG, occludin/zonulin IgA, occludin/zonulin IgM, lipopolysaccharide IgG, lipopolysaccharide IgA, and lipopolysaccharide IgM. That all sounds like something out of a science fiction novel, I know, but stick with me here. This is actually very interesting when you find out what zonulin and all those other things indicate.

Actomyosin antibodies appear in the blood in celiac disease, chronic hepatitis, autoimmune liver disorders, Crohn's disease, and myasthenia gravis. They also indicate autoimmunity against the gut. Occludin and zonulin are proteins in your gut that help hold the individual cells together and protect the body against invasion. When you have antibodies against these in your blood, it's another indicator of leaky gut as well as autoimmunity and celiac disease. The lipopolysaccharides are bacterial endotoxins that cause an immune response and inflammation in the gut. Lipopolysaccharides are bad news and are usually elevated in cases of depression, chronic fatigue, leaky gut, and dementia. So that's why you might choose the leaky gut test from Cyrex Labs. It can tell you information that would be scary enough to make you change your diet immediately—with no cheating.

If you are currently working with a functional medicine doctor who is well versed in testing for leaky gut, he or she should be able to order an intestinal permeability test for you. If you don't have a functional medicine doctor but would like to test yourself for leaky gut before embarking on the Paleo Autoimmune Protocol, I am currently available for one-on-one consultations via phone or Skype. Test kits can be mailed to you in the United States, Canada, and most international locations.

Another test you may want to consider before embarking on the Paleo Autoimmune Protocol is a food intolerance test that tests for IgG antibodies to a number of foods. This is different from a food allergy test, which tests for IgE antibodies to foods. One thing that happens when you have a leaky gut is that you start to develop multiple food sensitivities, characterized by IgG antibodies. Symptoms of an IgG reaction to a food, which can include headaches, fatigue, mood changes, sinusitis, joint pain, circles under the eyes, eczema, or gastric distress, can occur several hours to several days after you eat that food. This makes it difficult to pinpoint if you have a sensitivity to a particular food. On the other hand, an IgE reaction to a food is rather immediate and can include life-threatening and severe reactions such as swelling of the throat, tongue, face, and difficulty breathing.

An IgE reaction is what a conventional allergist will look for with a skin prick test.

Foods to Eliminate on the Paleo Autoimmune Protocol

Now let's get clear on the categories of foods that are eliminated on the Paleo Autoimmune Protocol. The list can seem daunting at first, but remember that this is only temporary to allow your gut to heal. You will be able to introduce MOST of the eliminated foods after strict adherence to the diet for six months. Some foods can be reintroduced after only 30 days.

Here's that list of foods you won't be eating for a while:

- Grains and pseudograins (wheat, rye, spelt, kamut, corn, oats, rice, teff, buckwheat, quinoa)
- Eggs (all types)
- Dairy (except for ghee and colostrum)
- Nuts (almonds, cashews, walnuts, pecans, macadamias, Brazil nuts, pistachios)
- Seeds (sesame, pumpkin, flax, sacha inchi, chia)
- Legumes (peanuts, beans, peas)
- Nightshades (eggplant, white potatoes, tomatoes, goji berries, bell peppers, hot peppers)
- *Coffee, tea, and Chocolate

- Seed-based and nightshade-based spices (black pepper, white pepper, curry, *cayenne, paprika, nutmeg, fennel, dill, celery seed, vanilla, and many others)
- ☆Starchy vegetables and tubers

I placed an asterisk on cayenne and coffee and a star on starchy vegetables and tubers because these foods are gray areas. Let me explain.

Cayenne is eliminated in most versions of the Paleo Autoimmune Protocol that you'll read about in other books. The reasoning is that cayenne is a nightshade. The nightshade family of vegetables and fruits (which includes peppers, potatoes, tomatoes, tobacco, and goji berries) is omitted from the Paleo Autoimmune Protocol because its members typically contain plant toxins that can be deadly in large amounts. Potatoes and tomatoes actually contain nicotine and can become highly addictive. Eating too many raw potatoes could actually kill you because you'd overdose on the plant toxin solanine. Small amounts of these plant poisons can worsen arthritis or induce headaches in some individuals. Chilies, cayenne, and habanero peppers, on the other hand, contain a plant chemical called capsaicin, which is what causes your mouth to burn when you eat them. Capsaicin is a protective mechanism of the plant, but it's actually not toxic to humans. Capsaicin has been highly researched as a plant medicine that can cause apoptosis (cell death) in cancer, alleviate pain, increase metabolic rate, and possibly even halt a variety of autoimmune diseases, including type 1 diabetes. Therefore, leaving hot peppers out of your diet may not provide any extra benefit, even though they are botanically in the nightshade family and typically omitted from the Paleo Autoimmune Protocol.

Next, coffee is eliminated from the Paleo Autoimmune Protocol because it is a seed and because it contains caffeine. Many people have adverse reactions to coffee either because they are caffeine-sensitive or they are consuming coffee that has been burned during the roasting or brewing process, has been contaminated with gluten, or contains mycotoxins. On the other hand, according to neurologist Dr. Perlmutter in *Brain Maker,* coffee can help heal a leaky gut by promoting a more favorable ratio of firmicutes bacteria to bacteroides bacteria in the gut. He actually recommends drinking three to five cups of coffee per day for optimal brain and gut health. Go to <u>energized.life/resources</u> for a list of coffee and other products I recommend.

That being said, if you have adrenal fatigue, you should avoid caffeine for at least 30 days. The proper test for adrenal fatigue involves at least four salivary samples throughout a 24-hour period. The adrenal hormones DHEA and cortisol follow a circadian rhythm, starting out high in the mornings and slowly dropping as the day progresses. At least that's what happens if your adrenal glands are functioning normally. Some individuals have exactly the opposite—low levels of cortisol in the morning and high cortisol at night. They have difficulty sleeping at night and difficulty getting out of bed in the morning. Other individuals have high cortisol all day, which usually results in excess belly fat and decreased muscle mass in the arms and legs. Still others will have low cortisol all the time. They're flat-out exhausted, with episodes of dizziness. Coffee would not be a good idea for any of these individuals with unhealthy adrenal glands. If you have a feeling your adrenal glands are out of whack, you can get 1-on-1 support from me via phone or Skype. We can test the circadian rhythm of cortisol and DHEA and then develop a personalized strategy based on your test results to get your circadian rhythm and adrenal health back to what it should be.

Before moving on to the next section of this book, I also want to touch briefly on the starchy vegetables. There's a controversy happening in the world of paleo concerning carbohydrates, of which I'm sure you're aware. You are probably wondering where I stand on the matter. We're talking specifically about the so-called "safe starches," which includes sweet potatoes, butternut squash, and white rice. Sweet potatoes and butternut squash are allowed on some versions of the Paleo Autoimmune Protocol diet because they are low in toxins and easy to digest.

However, most individuals with a leaky gut simply don't do well with starches. And this is the reason why I think beans and grains should also be avoided when you have a leaky gut or autoimmune condition. (Beans and grains are eliminated on the autoimmune protocol diet because they contain plant toxins. But all plants—including kale—contain some amount of toxins, so if you eliminated all foods that contain plant toxins you'd end up not eating plants at all.) Dr. Terry Wahls, who put her multiple sclerosis into remission, recommends eating nine cups of non-starchy vegetables per day in her book *The Wahls Protocol.* She and Dr. Perlmutter both recommend a ketogenic (low carb/high fat) diet for healing the gut and the brain. With a ketogenic diet, the body relies on fat instead of sugar as a primary fuel source. Although the jury is still out on exactly why some individuals simply can't tolerate the so-called "safe starches," I have a hunch that it has less to do with blood sugar and insulin directly, and more to do with the effect of starchy foods on our microbiome (the ecosystem of bacteria and yeast that live in our guts). Starchy foods feed the critters in our guts. If we have a leaky gut, autoimmune disease, or obesity, we've got too many bad guys living in our gut and not enough good guys. By eliminating starchy foods—including the "safe starches"—we can starve the bad guys and start to heal the gut. The reason why antibiotics only exacerbate the problem is that they often miss the target (overgrowth of particular species of bacteria that promote disease and obesity) and hit innocent bystanders (bacteria that protect us from disease and obesity) instead.

FODMAPs, SIBO, GAPS, SCD, and Keto...Oh My!

It's inevitable that if you're reading about the Paleo Autoimmune Protocol or simply looking for a grain-free pancake recipe online that you'll come across a bunch of acronyms and different nuances of the paleo-ish diet. It can all be extremely confusing and, in my opinion, the confusion can cause some individuals to end up with a bad case of orthorexia (an extreme preoccupation with avoiding foods perceived to cause real or imagined health problems). I want to explain all the acronyms briefly so that you won't stay awake all night wondering if you're going to die of SIBO or FODMAP poisoning.

Here's the deal. The bacteria that live in your gut thrive on carbohydrates—especially resistant starch, soluble fiber, and sugar. If you have small intestinal bacterial overgrowth (SIBO), foods that contain a lot of starches, soluble fibers, sugars, and FODMAPs can exacerbate your health problems by feeding species of bacteria that are already overly abundant. The purpose of all of these different acronym diets is to decrease your consumption of foods that feed the bacterial species that are causing gas and crowding out more-beneficial bacteria.

What exactly are FODMAPs? The acronym means Fermentable Oligosaccharides, Disaccharides, Monosaccharides, and Polyols. Basically, FODMAPs are short-chain carbohydrates. They are the type of carbohydrates that can cause some people to experience gas and an irritable bowel. The more infamous ones are beans, cabbage, onions, mushrooms, Brussels sprouts, and broccoli. There are very few fruits and vegetables that are low in FODMAPs. Much of the information about the Paleo Autoimmune Protocol you'll find online will also mention the FODMAPs.

By listening to your body, you will know if you have a problem with FODMAPs. Do you look nine months pregnant after eating an apple? Do you avoid beans in order to prevent social embarrassment? This is a sign that you have an overabundance of some of the mean bacteria that like to produce a lot of gas by fermenting some types of carbohydrates in your food. By eliminating starchy carbohydrates and restricting the amount of sugar in your diet for a few weeks, these rogue bacteria will die off. You'll be able to eat oodles of cabbage (and other foods high in FODMAPs) with no party-stopping consequences! (That is, if you wanted to eat oodles of cabbage.)

This is the idea behind the Specific Carbohydrate Diet (SCD) and the GAPS (Gut and Psychology Syndrome) diet. These each have their own protocols, but the basic idea is the same. By temporarily avoiding the foods that feed your intestinal bacteria, you cause pathogenic strains of bacteria to die. Then, you can reinoculate your gut with the appropriate strains of bacteria by taking probiotics. I believe this is one reason why some individuals thrive temporarily on a ketogenic diet that is inherently low in fermentable carbohydrates.

While you are doing the autoimmune protocol, you may want to reduce (not eliminate) foods high in FODMAPs unless you have a very severe reaction to them. Just use common sense. Don't eat onions, mushrooms, and an entire head of raw cabbage and then go on a date. I don't know anyone who would have good results from that.

Now here's a word of caution on ketogenic diets. In case you haven't already heard the ruckus, the quantity of carbohydrates required on the Paleo Autoimmune Protocol is an extremely controversial issue in the blogosphere. Some individuals don't do so well over the long term when they're consuming fewer than 50 grams of carbohydrates per day. Looking deeper into what these individuals are actually eating, it's often the case that they aren't eating any vegetables or fruits, they're eating poor-quality fats, and they're getting their calories from low-carb processed foods, soy products, and deli meats. I believe you should focus more on food quality, with an emphasis on non-starchy vegetables, naturally solid cooking fats, and wild meat and seafood. Many individuals achieve great results on 50 -100 grams of carbohydrates per day as long as they are eating enough fat to stay energized.

Okay, But What's for Dinner?

Now, after reading the extensive list of foods not allowed during the elimination phase of the Paleo Autoimmune Protocol, you might be feeling overwhelmed. You might be thinking this is some kind of starvation diet. Perhaps you aren't interested in going hungry for six months, avoiding your favorite foods, missing out on social events, and losing weight from an already fragile frame. When you read the list of all the foods you CAN'T have, it can seem at first like there's nothing left. What will your life be like without chocolate, bread, pasta, almond butter, and goji berries?!

The truth is that doing the Paleo Autoimmune Protocol can actually be a lot of fun when you know how to *actually* do it. Staying up late at night reading blog posts, clicking links, asking questions on Facebook and online forums, and trying to find Paleo Autoimmune Protocol recipes for everything you're used to eating (waffles, toaster pastries, birthday cake, enchiladas, pizza, ice cream, sandwiches, etc.) is NOT the way to succeed on the Paleo Autoimmune Protocol.

Yes, it's great to have those resources. And it can be fun to learn how to make "familiar" foods using new ingredients. I'm not against learning how to make a birthday cake free of grains, eggs, and refined sugar. If you enjoy spending lots of time in the kitchen or entertaining guests with novel recipes, then I highly recommend spending some time on Pinterest or your favorite Paleo Autoimmune Protocol food blogs to find different recipes to try for special occasions.

But when it comes right down to it, to succeed on the Paleo Autoimmune Protocol, you aren't going to be making Paleo Autoimmune Protocol breakfast crepes with fruit compote for breakfast on Monday, Paleo Autoimmune Protocol waffles for breakfast on Tuesday, Paleo Autoimmune Protocol breakfast cereal on Wednesday, and so on for every single meal for the next six months. Unless you're a professional chef who spends eight hours in the kitchen every day, that's a guaranteed way to go absolutely crazy after about a week!

In order to *actually* do the Paleo Autoimmune Protocol, the first thing you need to do is get your family on board. Ideally, all food ingredients and meals made inside your home should be foods that are "allowed" on the autoimmune protocol. One reason for this is that cross-contamination can occur, especially if you're cooking a "special" meal for yourself while you're cooking spaghetti and meatballs for your husband and children. Sharing the same dishes and cooking vessels can be another obstacle. What if your husband cooks his grilled cheese sandwich in the iron skillet that you normally use for your breakfast stir-fries? If your family insists upon having non-Paleo Autoimmune Protocol foods inside the home, then you should at least agree to have separate cookware for Paleo Autoimmune Protocol foods only. This is one of the best ways to protect against accidental exposure to foods that you are temporarily eliminating.

Next, you should be prepared to start preparing and cooking the majority of your meals at home. While it is certainly possible to eat at restaurants when you are on the Paleo Autoimmune Protocol, you should not rely on restaurant fare as a quick meal when you don't have time to cook. Unless you happen to have a Paleo Autoimmune Protocol restaurant near your home or workplace, eating at restaurants should be for social occasions only. You might actually have to eat your meal before going to the restaurant and then order a plain salad. Depending on the type of restaurant you're going to, you might be able to speak to the chef before you go, explain that you have medical dietary restrictions, and request an off-menu meal. A vegetable plate with a baked sweet potato and wild-caught fish can often be had.

So how are you going to prepare nearly all of your meals at home? This is almost unheard of in today's hectic world where the majority of people don't even take the time to sit down at the table to eat. Perhaps you are one of the many individuals who skip breakfast, grab some donuts on the way to work, improvise a lunch by grabbing something from a nearby fast food restaurant, and then cook something out of a box at dinner. Cooking absolutely everything from scratch can seem like something you simply don't have time for.

I'm here to tell you the surprising news that you've been waiting to hear. With a little planning—and taking action on that planning—you can easily prepare all your meals for the week on a Sunday afternoon. You'll need to get some stainless steel or glass food storage containers to store your meals, and you'll need to have some quality cookware to cook with. And you'll need to block off about four hours of time each week (I recommend Sunday afternoons) for the process. Then you will be set up for success on the Paleo Autoimmune Protocol.

Now what kinds of things are you going to be eating on the AIP? Is there anything actually left to eat when you eliminate the major food groups of French fries, burritos, pizza, chocolate, and nut butter? The answer is yes! Except for the nightshades, just about every fruit and vegetable is a free-for-all. I'm talking about kale, spinach, chard, lettuce, cauliflower, broccoli, cabbage, rutabaga, radishes, turnips, onions, squash, pumpkin, mushrooms, beets, carrots, sweet potatoes, okra, collards, garlic, artichokes, apples, oranges, grapefruits, coconuts, mangos, pineapples, papayas, kiwis, figs, dates, peaches, plums, pears, strawberries, blueberries, blackberries, grapes, lychees, mulberries, acai berries, and more! Another free-for-all is grass-fed meat, antibiotic-free poultry, and wild-caught fish and seafood. That includes beef, bison (buffalo), ostrich, venison, duck, chicken, turkey, rabbit, trout, tuna, salmon, sardines, herring, crab, shrimp, lobster, oysters, clams, mussels, organ meats, caviar, bone broth, and several others.

There are more foods that you CAN eat on the AIP than those you CAN'T eat. I bet you'll have a much more interesting and varied diet than anyone you know who has no *conscious* dietary restrictions. (Most people on a processed food diet actually only eat the same ten foods over and over without realizing it: corn, wheat, eggs, potatoes, tomatoes, milk, meat, soy, peanuts, and cottonseeds.)

Now, after reading the list of allowed foods, you may be thinking, "There's no way I'm eating a can of tuna fish and a can of spinach for breakfast. This sounds like a disgusting diet! And what's for lunch? A bowl of grapes and chicken liver?" Barf! In no way am I suggesting that you're going to be confined to gross and unappetizing meals! The Paleo Autoimmune Protocol is not an exercise in self-torture or missing out on the everyday pleasure of eating delicious and enticing food. And it's certainly not an exercise in going hungry.

If you are going to *actually* do the Paleo Autoimmune Protocol, you are going to have to start with ingredients that taste good. This means buying fresh vegetables and sustainably raised meats whenever possible. Canned and frozen vegetables are often flavorless and lacking in desirable texture unless you do your own canning and freezing. Oftentimes, even fresh vegetables and fruits are wilted and lifeless if they have been transported many miles from where they were grown and then stored on grocery shelves for days or weeks. Seek out fresh, locally grown fruits and vegetables at a local farmer's market and only buy grocery store produce that looks fresh and vibrant in color. This makes a huge difference in how your food is going to taste. If cost is truly an issue, you may be able to work something out with a local farmer. Ask for the bruised or "ugly" crops that can't be sold but are just as tasty and nutrient-dense as the more attractive part of the harvest that goes to the market. Some individuals even choose to start growing some of their own organic produce.

The quality of your meat also plays an important role in how it's going to taste without all the typical food additives that are used by the food companies to get you addicted to a processed food product. A chicken breast from a sick factory-farmed chicken that was fed antibiotics and genetically modified corn and never saw the light of day is not going to taste good if you try to bake it in the oven or leave it in a crockpot with an onion and a carrot. If you read the label closely for a raw chicken, you'll likely notice that it has been injected with a saline solution and "natural flavors" of unknown origin. That's really pretty gross. Don't waste your money on that, and definitely don't force yourself or your family to try to eat it. The only way to make that taste good is to slather it with Velveeta cheese or deep-fry it in flour and lard. Just don't.

The absolute best way to go about getting good quality meat is to buy a second freezer or at least clean all the junk out of the freezer you already have. Then check your local farmer's market or look online at eatwild.com for a local farmer who feeds their animals a species-appropriate diet, doesn't use growth hormones, and doesn't medicate their animals with antibiotics for the purpose of making them fat or as a way to make up for crowded and unsanitary living conditions. Then buy your meat in bulk, including the "odd bits" such as the organs and bones. This is actually a little money-saving tip that will allow you to eat well even on a budget. The price per pound for grass-fed beef or pasture-raised chicken might be more than what you'd pay for conventionally raised meat at the grocery store, but you also won't be flushing money down the toilet in the form of processed convenience foods, restaurant fare, antacids, and over-the-counter pain relievers.

Now I know that many of the individuals who read this book are simply not going to buy a big ole freezer and then fill it with half a cow and a few chickens. Perhaps you are one of those individuals who are simply saying, "That's not happening." You might live in a small space and prefer not to have a cow in your closet. I get it! Or perhaps you just don't live in an area where there's an abundance of small family farms raising happy animals that graze on organic green grass and bugs. You might be surrounded by fields of genetically modified corn. Or you might live in a literal food desert. There is still an option for you. Get your grass-fed meat delivered in the mail. This is what I did during one stage of my journey with this Paleo Autoimmune Protocol thing, and it was great. Getting food in the mail is a lot of fun. You can order grass-fed beef, duck, chicken, bone broth, pemmican, jerky, bacon, and other great-quality meats from the company that I use by going to energized.life/resources.

If you want to *actually* do the Paleo Autoimmune Protocol, you will also need to eat fish. But wait! Before you turn up your nose and think there's no way you're going to become a fish eater, please hear me out. High-quality, toxin-free fish and seafood is one of the key components of the Paleo Autoimmune Protocol for healing a leaky gut, getting rid of chronic inflammation and brain fog, regulating your immune system, and putting your autoimmune disease into remission. You need at least twelve ounces of fatty fish or shellfish per week. This means you'll need to be eating wild salmon, tuna belly, sardines, herring, and/or oysters three times per week. You can access a good clean source of fish and seafood by going to energized.life/resources. If you're a fish hater, you might want to start out with a product such as the wild salmon pieces or the manila clams. I always have a stockpile of sardines and mackerel in my pantry, although I don't care for the mushy texture of most canned fish products that are collecting dust on grocery shelves. I also love the seared Albacore and the skin-on salmon fillets I get online because in the area where I live, all the salmon is farm-raised. (Farm-raised salmon is something to avoid because it is chock full of pro-inflammatory fats due to being raised on genetically modified soy and corn instead of a species-appropriate diet of small fish and phytoplankton.)

How much meat, poultry, and fish are you going to be eating on the Paleo Autoimmune Protocol? Everyone out there in cyberspace seems to have a different opinion about how much protein the human body needs. To put it simply, the amount of protein your body needs to stay alive is much less than the amount of protein your body needs to thrive. And it's usually best to space your protein intake throughout the day instead of getting your protein all in one meal. That's because your body can't store protein. If you just eat a giant steak for breakfast, your body is going to end up turning part of that steak into sugar and burning it as energy (or storing it as fat). Usually, a four-ounce portion of meat, poultry, fish, or shellfish is a good amount for a meal, and eight to twelve ounces is an ideal amount for the entire day.

So by now we've gone over how to get fruits and vegetables that don't taste like watery Styrofoam, how to get meat and poultry that isn't causing planetary destruction, and where to buy fish that doesn't reek like a bad case of candida. What's next? What else are you going to be eating on the Paleo Autoimmune Protocol?

Fats That Heal vs. Fats That Kill

Fat. Yep, I said it. On this "diet," you will be putting fat on your food. This is a concept that seems absolutely crazy to the generation of individuals who grew up during the 80s and 90s. Those were the decades in which obesity truly reached "epidemic" proportions, and every time we turned on the TV or picked up a newspaper or magazine there was something about how the fat on our food was turning us into Hansel & Gretel. Except no one ever pointed out, that according to the classic children's fairy tale, Hansel & Gretel were fattened up with candies and sweets, not boluses of butter, lard, and coconut oil. But keep in mind that this was before the internet. Any challenge to the prevailing low-fat Holy Grail that was going to save us all from getting fat simply didn't get a soundbite on Oprah or the evening news.

But now the truth is out on fat. Anyone who has ever seen the viral *Time* magazine cover that proclaims "Eat Butter" has now been made aware that America didn't have a weight problem during the days in which butter was added to pretty much everything. And those skinny French women who are buying up the size 00 jeans on the mannequins in the window of Bloomingdale's? They're buying up all the butter too!

If you've already read blogs and books on the Paleo Autoimmune Protocol, you probably already know this stuff. But just in case you're one of the millions of consumers out there who is keeping Snackwell's and Pam in business (or not yet convinced that fat is safe to eat), I want to explain the difference between fat that kills and fat that heals.

Fats that are *naturally* solid at room temperature or when cooled, such as butter, ghee (clarified butter), lard (rendered pork fat), tallow (rendered beef fat), schmaltz (rendered poultry fat), coconut oil, and palm kernel oil, contain more saturated fatty acids than fats that are liquid even when refrigerated. Despite widespread belief since World War II that naturally saturated fatty acids cause cancer and heart disease, there's absolutely no scientific evidence to back up this claim. Don't take my word for it. See this article in The New York Times, spend an afternoon investigating the scientific literature, and if you still aren't convinced, you might want to read *Death By Food Pyramid*.

The truth is that there were shortages of several different foods during the war, and US citizens had to ration their usage of those foods. Rationed food included sugar, butter, bacon, coffee, eggs, cheese, and meat. Margarine, a cheap substitute for butter that was made out of hydrogenated vegetable oil, had been invented in the early 1900s. It tasted horrible and had an unappealing white color. To make matters worse for the margarine manufacturers, it was illegal to add yellow food dye to margarine because it might fool consumers into thinking they were buying real butter. But when butter came into short supply in 1942, margarine was marketed as "Victory Spread." Housewives began buying margarine as a symbol of their patriotism and also as a way to deal with the butter rationing. It was also during this time that a variety of government-funded studies began to show that butter, bacon, eggs, cheese, and meat contributed to heart disease; margarine was presented as the healthy alternative.

But in fact, the reverse was true. The rising incidence of heart disease could be directly attributed to the increase in consumption of margarine. This is not only because of the fatty acid composition of the vegetable oils used to make margarine, but also due to the unique process that changes a liquid oil into a solid one. To make the vegetable oils solid at room temperature for shelf-stable products like crackers, cookies, breads, and breakfast cereals, the food manufacturers figured out how to add hydrogen to turn an unsaturated vegetable oil into a saturated fat. No one realized at the time that hydrogenation—artificially adding hydrogen atoms to an unsaturated vegetable oil—changes the configuration of hydrogen atoms in the unsaturated fat to a "trans" position that is not found in nature and that is harmful to the human body. Sure, there are some naturally occurring trans fats (known as vaccenic acid) in meat and dairy from ruminant animals, but it has a different fatty acid profile than industrial trans fats and has been associated with reduced incidence of heart disease, diabetes, and obesity. I'm not making this stuff up! You can read more about this here http://www.ncbi.nlm.nih.gov/pubmed/25534067 and here http://jn.nutrition.org/content/140/1/18.

The hydrogenated vegetable oils that replaced naturally saturated fats didn't taste as good as animal fats, but they were a lot cheaper. Crisco (vegetable "shortening") replaced lard and tallow as a solid fat for baking and frying. Margarine replaced butter as a fat for enhancing the flavor of potatoes, vegetables, cookies, and breads. At first, people were reluctant to switch to these cheaper fats because of the taste.

The food manufacturers had to come up with a way to sell them. They funded a bunch of "research" studies to "prove" that vegetable oils are healthier than animal fats, and you probably know the results of that. Our government, our medical schools, and concerned home cooks all hopped on board that wagon.

The take-home lesson here is that the fats that are naturally solid at room temperature were used in cooking long before the post-WWII explosion of cancer, heart disease, diabetes, and obesity. These fats make your food more pleasurable to the taste and more satiating. Replacing these naturally occurring, stable fats with vegetable oils not only makes your food less delicious and satisfying (therefore causing you to eat more because you aren't feeding it the rich animal-based fats it's craving), but it also leads to a grab bag of "modern diseases" due to the presence of never-before-found-in-nature trans fats.

Each of the naturally solid cooking fats has its own unique characteristics and benefits to the human body. I think it's important for everyone with a body to understand the benefits of these fats that have been vilified by crony capitalists and mostly eliminated from the food supply over the past fifty years. (Even the tub of white stuff labeled "lard" in some grocery stores is not real lard.)

Coconut and palm kernel oil are high in lauric acid, a type of saturated fatty acid that has a 12-carbon atom chain and is thus recognized as a medium-chain fatty acid. This special fat raises your level of high-density lipoproteins, which are regarded as protective against atherosclerosis (heart disease). Another benefit of medium-chain triglycerides in general is that they promote fat oxidation and reduced food intake, meaning they cause you to burn fat for energy and also unconsciously eat less food. Unlike other types of fats, they don't require bile for digestion, and they are easily absorbed and used for energy. Therefore, they tend to be good for people with malabsorption problems. There are also numerous studies with promising results concerning the benefits of medium-chain tryiglycerides for people with epilepsy, Parkinson's, and Alzheimer's.

Tallow, lard, and schmaltz contain significant amounts of stearic acid, depending on what the animals they come from were fed. Stearic acid is less likely to be incorporated into cholesterol esters than some other types of fatty acids, and they're associated with lowered numbers of low-density lipoproteins.

Butter and ghee are particularly high in butyric acid, which is also an end product of the fermentation process of anaerobic bacteria. Therefore, butyric acid is also found in kombucha tea. The health benefits are numerous and well studied, although none of this has been publicized on a TV near you. Butyric acid inhibits the growth of colon cancer cells and promotes the growth of healthy epithelial cells of the colon. It's therefore extremely beneficial for promoting the healing process for leaky gut and other health problems of the colon. Many individuals also notice that including butter or ghee in their diet gives their skin a healthier glow.

Unfortunately, butter and ghee are eliminated from the strictest version of the Paleo Autoimmune Protocol. This is because some individuals with an autoimmune disease can have reactions to even the small amounts of lactose and casein that may be present in these fats. An IgG antibody test should be able to provide you with some indication of whether you are sensitive to any components of dairy. In the case of butter and ghee, if in doubt, leave it out.

Now let's move on to the topic of fats that are regarded as essential fatty acids. They're called "essential" because our bodies require them for good health, but we can't synthesize them on our own. All of them are very fragile, and therefore are not suitable for use as cooking oils. (But guess what the Big Food manufacturers did with them?) These fragile fats include alpha-linolenic acid (ALA), linoleic acid (LA), docosahexaenoic acid (DHA), eicosapentaenoic acid (EPA), and gamma linolenic acid (GLA). These words can sound like a bunch of confusing chemistry gobbledygook, so I'm going to go over each one briefly below.

ALA is known as an omega-3 fatty acid, meaning it has a double bond at the third carbon atom from the end of its carbon chain. It's a powerful anti-inflammatory agent that is also a building block for our cell membranes. When we have the right amount of it, our cells are happy. If we're deficient in it, on the other hand, we can suffer from aches, pains, mental health disorders, dermatitis, and chronic health conditions associated with inflammation. The most abundant sources of ALA are chia seeds, flax seeds, hemp seeds, and walnuts, which are all foods that are eliminated on the Paleo Autoimmune Protocol. The good news is that ALA is present in small amounts in most vegetables, grass-fed meat, and poultry that was fed ALA-rich seeds. There's no widespread consensus on how much ALA we need, but I believe that number to be at least 1–2 grams per day.

LA is a type of omega-6 fatty acid with its carbon atom on the sixth carbon from the end of its carbon chain. It competes with ALA as a building block for our cell membranes. And in contrast to ALA, LA is pro-inflammatory. This is useful for promoting growth and cell repair after exercise or injury. A proper balance between ALA and LA in our diets is crucial for good health. We need both, but most people are getting far too much LA and are therefore suffering the consequence of chronic inflammation everywhere in their bodies at all times. This is because LA is abundant in so many foods in the modern diet—especially corn oil and meat from corn-fed animals. The ratio of ALA to LA is much more balanced in grass-fed meats, which is why you should be choosing those meats where possible. And please remember this: friends don't let friends cook with corn oil.

Next, we have DHA and EPA. These fats are only present in algae, phytoplankton, fish, and shellfish. They're both omega-3 fatty acids, though they have different functions in the body. DHA is the main ingredient in the brain, cerebral cortex, retina of the eyes, skin, and men's testicles and sperm. A deficiency of DHA is associated with cognitive decline, mood disorders, Alzheimer's, Parkinson's, decreased visual acuity, infertility, psoriasis, cancer, and autoimmune disease. EPA, on the other hand, has the role of preventing blood clots and inflammation. Some studies suggest that EPA may be helpful in treating schizophrenia and depression, as well as any condition associated with chronic inflammation.

GLA is an omega-6 fatty acid that can be produced from LA in a healthy person with no nutritional deficiencies. GLA plays a role in regulation of the immune system and also in skin health, so if you have an autoimmune condition, it's probably best to get some GLA in your diet rather than rely on your body's ability to convert LA into GLA.

Now by this point you may be wondering where olive oil fits into this picture. And what about avocados and avocado oil? Both of these flavorful plant-based fats are high in oleic acid, which is a monounsaturated omega-9 fatty acid. This particular type of fatty acid is not required by the body, although it does have some interesting characteristics. All animals on the planet release oleic acid from their bodies when they die, causing corpses to have a characteristic odor.

Also, in individuals with severe deficiencies in essential fatty acids, either from fat malabsorption or from a strict vegan diet, the body will convert oleic acid into mead acid. Mead acid is a polyunsaturated omega-9 acid that inhibits bone formation. Therefore, one could reason that a deficiency in any of the essential fatty acids (ALA, LA, DHA, EPA, and GLA) will eventually lead to short stature in children and osteoporosis in adults. I strongly suspect that the health benefits of olive oil and avocados are more related to the polyphenols, antioxidants, and other phytochemicals found in these foods. The body requires fats in order to absorb phytochemicals as well as vitamins (even the so-called "water-soluble" ones), and olives and avocados are two of the only edible fruits on the planet that provide a rich source of fats to enable efficient absorption of their nutrients.

Recently, there has been an increase of interest in the use of safflower oil, which is a rich source of linoleic and oleic acid. It's often sold as a weight-loss supplement because of a 16-week study at Ohio State University that showed that safflower oil helped post-menopausal women with high blood sugar to lose belly fat. However, another study found that replacing animal fats with safflower oil actually increased risk of death from all causes. Subsequent studies have found that while safflower oil can decrease total cholesterol level, it actually increases death by heart disease. There are definitely other ways to lose belly fat that won't increase your risk of death! Following the Paleo Autoimmune Protocol as outlined in this book is a great way to start. Plenty of research suggests that a leaky gut is what contributes to belly fat in the first place.

So what does this all mean for you if you're going to actually do the Paleo Autoimmune Protocol? Basically, it's the quality and variety of fats on your plate every day that is going to play a crucial role in whether or not the Paleo Autoimmune Protocol works for you. Use stable cooking fats from clean, grass-fed sources, and make sure you're eating fatty fish three times a week. Just remember that simple take-away message and you have a good chance of supplying your body with an adequate amount of essential fatty acids in the right ratios.

That being said, I have found it to be very helpful to test for fatty acid deficiencies using a simple bloodspot test. While it's common for most people to have an excessive amount of omega-6 fatty acids in relation to omega-3 fatty acids in their cell membranes (thus promoting a pro-inflammatory state), some health-conscious individuals can end up consuming an adequate amount of omega-3 fatty acids and not enough omega-6 fatty acids. This can cause a variety of symptoms, including mental disturbances, behavior changes, hair loss, eczema, infertility, frequent miscarriages, frequent infections, immune dysregulation, and other "mysterious" problems despite eating a "perfect" diet. What if you could resolve these symptoms for yourself, simply by objectively measuring your fatty acids and figuring out which ones are out of balance? You can set up a phone or Skype appointment with me if you would like to do a fatty acid bloodspot test to find out how you are doing in regard to eating the right variety and amounts of fatty acids. I will provide you with one-on-one guidance on what you need to eat in order to fix your fatty acid imbalance.

By now, you should be reasonably clear on what kinds of foods you should be eating on the Paleo Autoimmune Protocol. You're aware that you'll need to start buying fresh fruits and vegetables—locally grown and pesticide-free when possible. The quality of your meat, poultry, and fish is extremely important. Grass-fed and pasture-raised is best because this is going to provide you with a healthier fatty acid profile than animals that were raised on genetically modified corn and Hershey's chocolate bars. Animals that are allowed to roam around and eat a species-appropriate diet will also have a better flavor and texture. (This is also why some individuals will go through extraordinary efforts to procure wild game instead of just going to the grocery store to buy some hamburger meat.) When purchasing fish, always choose wild-caught because this is going to provide you with the essential fatty acids required by your brain, eyes, and nervous system.

And after all the chatter about fats, by now you should understand that all the essential fatty acids needed by the body are available in fats of animal origin. As long as you're eating fish, grass-fed meats, butter, tallow, and lard, you should be getting all the fats that your body can't make on its own. If you're trying to rely on plant-based fats only, or if you're avoiding any fat in your diet, you will eventually run into trouble and probably start making large amounts of mead acid, which can prove deleterious to your bones.

How to Take Action

Now let's talk about how to actually implement the information in this book. It's one thing to know which foods to eliminate for 30 days and how to find quality foods in a grocery store, farmer's market, or online; it's an entirely different ballgame when it comes to actually doing it. Simply knowing how to do something doesn't translate into actually getting started and sticking with it even when you don't feel like it. It's so easy to think to oneself, "I'll start this tomorrow." Then if you ever get started on the Paleo Autoimmune Protocol, there will always be some life circumstance that could derail you. Your husband brings home pizza, there's a birthday party or a wedding to attend, you're stuck in an airport and you're "hangry," or you come home from work and you're too tired to cook.

There's a way to do the Paleo Autoimmune Protocol that doesn't rely on your willpower to resist the pizza or cake, or your ability to slave over a hot stove to produce three gourmet Paleo Autoimmune Protocol meals per day. And you don't have to survive on canned tuna and broccoli every day—or ever. Enter the art of meal planning, shopping like a PRO, and batch cooking.

Meal planning can be as simple or elaborate as you want to make it. You may want to make a spreadsheet of your meals for the week, print it out, and post it on your refrigerator. For some ideas on what to cook, you might look through some of your favorite Paleo Autoimmune Protocol cookbooks. (I've listed a few of my favorites at energized.life/resources. If you're already good at improvising your own recipes based on a few simple ingredients, you won't necessarily have to follow a recipe for each meal. Just figure out what you want to eat for your next 21 meals. I recommend doing this on a Saturday, or the first day of your weekend. You need to have at least 12 ounces of fish (per person per week), between 2–3 pounds of meat or poultry (per person per week), 5–9 servings of non-starchy vegetables (per person per day), 1 serving of berries (per person per day), plenty of solid cooking fats such as coconut oil and lard, a variety of spices for flavoring your food, and some pantry staples such as coconut flour for baking or to use as a thickener in soups and gravies.

If you're just getting started, you may have to empty any processed foods from your freezer, throw away condiments that contain high-fructose corn syrup and chemical additives, and totally empty your pantry. The Campbell's soups, Rice-a-Roni, Kraft Macaroni & Cheese, "gluten-free" breakfast cereal, granola bars, peanut butter, cookies, crackers, and other things of that nature will have to go. If you can get these foods out of your kitchen, they'll be far less likely to end up on your plate.

Make a list of the items you need to get to make your next 21 meals. If you've ordered your meat, poultry, and fish in bulk and established a pantry full of coconut flour, spices, and cooking fats, you'll only need to buy fresh fruits and vegetables on a weekly basis. This can be done with a trip to the farmer's market if you have an active market in your area.

There will be times when you'll have to go to a grocery store, however, and this is something that can be difficult when you intend to only buy Paleo Autoimmune Protocol foods. Whether you're at a Whole Foods or a Walmart Supercenter, there are many things that can go wrong. You may walk down an aisle to get coconut butter and carob to make healthy treats, but suddenly some almond butter and baking chocolate "falls" off the shelf and lands in your cart. These ingredients aren't Paleo Autoimmune Protocol, but they're technically paleo...right? This would surely be tasty with a dollop of ice cream, wouldn't it? Down the freezer aisle, the gluten-free ice cream is placed strategically next to the gluten-free pizza. All these things just start hopping into your basket. Then by the time you get to the checkout, you realize you've blown your budget as well as your entire meal plan. You're stuck with junk food for the rest of the week.

I know this is one of the toughest things when you're starting out because I've been there. Eleven years ago, when I was trying to transition from vegan to paleo, the sprouted grain bread and organic vegan blueberry bran muffins just kept ending up in my cart. "Just one last piece of toast and one more vegan blueberry muffin," I kept telling myself. Then the chocolate soy ice cream was always right next to the sprouted grain bread and bran muffins. It, too, would somehow magically end up in my cart. What pairs nicely with a pint of chocolate faux ice cream? Vegan Italian food chock full of tofu and wheat gluten, of course! It was a vicious cycle until I figured out a system that would prevent my lizard brain from leaping for its addictions. Now that I'm no longer addicted to wheat and soy, it doesn't appeal to me at all. You could take me to a "healthy" bakery and I wouldn't be fazed.

The system I figured out is what I call shopping like a PRO, which is an acronym to help you remember what to do when you walk through the grocery store doors. The "P" stands for perimeter or produce. The first item in your shopping cart should be a produce item—ideally a non-starchy vegetable such as a fresh cauliflower or artichoke. This is a little "psychological" hack. Your brain will unconsciously start seeking out items to match the first item you put in your cart. Suddenly you're reaching for parsley, blueberries, lemons, and kale because these all match the cauliflower and artichoke. (This phenomenon is also why if the first item you put in your cart is a "treat," you'll unconsciously start reaching for more treats to match the first one.) Next, the "R" stands for refrigerated. If you're out of meat, poultry, or fish, go to the refrigerated section and get the best quality proteins available. Finally, the "O" stands for other. Are you out of butter? Need more coconut flour for your planned breakfast on Tuesday morning? Go to the appropriate aisle now, and only get the items on your list. Then get out of the store, because next up is batch cooking.

I suggest doing your batch cooking on a Sunday, or the day after your shopping day. Set aside at least four hours to rinse and chop veggies and cook your meats for the week. This may sound a little overwhelming at first, but it saves time and is actually a lot easier than trying to cook every day or when you're already hungry.

Here's an example of how to batch cook. You might plan on having baked wild salmon for lunch on Monday, Wednesday, and Friday, chicken for lunch on Tuesday, Thursday, and Saturday, and bison sausage for your breakfasts. Simply get all those ingredients out and cook them. While the meats are baking in the oven or cooking in the slow cooker, you can be chopping, steaming, or sautéing your veggies. Then store your cooked meals in a sealable glass or stainless steel container in the refrigerator. It's a good idea to label each container to identify what's in it, when you cooked it, and when you plan to eat it based on your week's menu.

Your 1-Week Meal Plan with Recipes

In this chapter, you'll find a sample 1-week meal plan with recipes for some of the menu items that aren't as easy to improvise. For the other menu items, just start with fresh ingredients and heat them in a pan, slow cooker, or oven with a little bit of solid cooking fat and your favorite spices. If you tend to burn everything you cook or are prone to "kitchen accidents" involving your local fire department, go with the slow cooker. You can throw just about anything in there, set it on low, come back eight hours later, and have a hot meal. For a list of high-quality ingredients, supplements, meal delivery services, and cooking classes I recommend, go to <u>energized.life/resources</u>.

Sample 1-Week Meal Plan

Sunday

- Breakfast: Smoked Wild Alaskan Sockeye Salmon with Avocado and Fennel Salad
- Lunch: Cauliflower, Carrots, and Green Beans Stir-Fried in Ghee
- Dinner: Bunless Bison Burgers with Lettuce, Sautéed Onions, and Mushrooms
- Dessert: Blackberry Colostrum Ice Cream

Monday

- Breakfast: Turkey and Sage Sausage Scramble with Veggies and Coconut Oil
- Lunch: Chicken Thighs, Pureed Cauliflower with Ghee, Romaine Lettuce, Steamed Beets
- Dinner: Veggie Stir-Fry with Red Boat Fish Sauce and Coconut Oil
- Dessert: Mango with Lime and Sea Salt

Tuesday

- Breakfast: Liver Pâté with Celery, Carrot, and Beet Dipping Sticks
- Lunch: Bunless Bison Burgers, Pureed Cauliflower with Ghee, Stir-Fried Green Beans
- Dinner: Tuscan-Style Steamed Clams with Roasted Artichoke
- Dessert: Coconut Carob Colostrum Energy Balls

Wednesday

- Breakfast: Crockpot Chicken Stew with Carrots, Celery, and Onions
- Lunch: Sardines with Avocado, Beets, and Fennel
- Dinner: Steamed Veggies with Ghee and Coconut Flakes
- Dessert: Homemade Gelatin Gummies

Thursday

- Breakfast: Colostrum Pancakes, Salmon Bacon, and Berry Compote
- Lunch: Crockpot Chicken Stew
- Dinner: Grass-Fed Steak, Pureed Cauliflower with Ghee, Heirloom Carrots
- Dessert: Carob Avocado Mousse

Friday

- Breakfast: Turkey and Sage Sausage with Veggie Stir-Fry in Coconut Oil
- Lunch: Ahi Tuna Carpaccio with Red Onion & Parsley
- Dinner: Steamed Beets and Greens Drizzled in Olive Oil
- Dessert: Strawberry-Apple Pie with Coconut Lard Crust

Saturday

- Breakfast: Recovery Smoothie (Pure Paleo Protein, Frozen Berries, PaleoGreens, MCT Oil, Ice)
- Lunch: Shrimp Spring Rolls with Coconut Wrap
- Snack: Sliced Mango with Lime and Sea Salt
- Dinner: Buddha's Delight Stir-Fry in Coconut Oil

RECIPES

Blackberry Colostrum Ice Cream (Makes 2 Servings)

- 16 oz frozen organic raspberries
- 4 Tbsp colostrum
- 2 Tbsp ghee
- liquid stevia
- small amount of water

Blend all ingredients in a Vitamix or blender. Serve in a ceramic heart bowl.

Liver Pâté

- 1 lb grass-fed beef liver
- 6 slices pasture-raised bacon
- 1 medium onion
- 3 cloves garlic
- 8 Tbsp grass-fed ghee
- 1 Tbsp dried sage
- sea salt

Add all ingredients except ghee to a slow cooker. Cook on the lowest setting for 8 hours. Then add to a food processor with ghee and puree until smooth.

Colostrum Pancakes (Makes 1 Serving)

- ¼ cup coconut flour
- 2 Tbsp colostrum
- ¼ cup mashed avocado
- 1 banana
- small amount of water

Mix all ingredients evenly. Spoon onto an iron skillet with coconut oil or ghee. Cook for approximately 2 minutes on each side.

Coconut Carob Colostrum Energy Balls (Makes 2 Servings)

- 2 Tbsp coconut butter
- 2 Tbsp coconut flakes
- 1 Tbsp raw honey
- 2 tsp carob powder
- 2 tsp colostrum

Mix all ingredients and shape into balls. Store in refrigerator or freezer.

Homemade Gelatin Gummies

- 16 oz fresh-pressed juice
- 8 Tbsp grass-fed gelatin
- 6 tsp Vitamin C powder

Combine all ingredients and heat until almost boiling. Transfer to a glass or stainless steel gelatin mold. Refrigerate until jelled.

Strawberry-Apple Pie

Crust Ingredients:

- 2 Tbsp lard
- 1 banana, mashed
- ¾ cup coconut flour
- 2 tsp cinnamon
- pinch of sea salt

Optional: Double this recipe for a top crust. You could also use coconut flakes as your pie topping.

Crust Directions:

1. Preheat oven to 400 degrees.
2. In a mixing bowl, mash lard, banana, cinnamon, and salt together with a fork.
3. Add coconut flour and stir until you reach a doughy consistency.
4. Transfer dough to a 9-inch pie plate and use your hands to mash dough into an even crust.
5. Prick dough with a fork.

6. Bake for 10 minutes or until lightly brown. Remove from oven and cool.

Filling Ingredients:

- 2 pints fresh strawberries, sliced
- 1 large tart apple
- ¼ cup coconut flour
- ⅓ cup stevia leaf powder
- 1 tsp cinnamon
- 1 pinch sea salt
- 2 Tbsp MCT oil or ghee
- Optional: 1 dropperful of chaga extract

Filling Directions:

1. Preheat oven to 375 F.
2. Combine coconut flour, stevia powder, cinnamon, and sea salt in a mixing bowl.
3. Add in the strawberries and apple and stir well.
4. Place the mixture into the pie shell.
5. Drizzle with Brain Octane or melted ghee.
6. Add top crust or coconut flakes if you want your pie to have a "lid" instead of being open-faced.
7. Bake for 40 minutes or until done throughout.

Recovery Smoothie

- 2 Tbsp grass-fed beef collagen protein powder
- 1 scoop mint PaleoGreens
- 1 Tbsp MCT Colada
- 1 Tbsp Colostrum
- 1.5 cups frozen berries
- water or ice

Blend all ingredients in a blender and serve in a tall glass.

Recommended Supplements

In order to receive the best results with the Paleo Autoimmune Protocol, I also recommend taking a few supplements. Now I know that the caveman didn't take nutritional supplements, but he also didn't suffer from chronic leaky gut syndrome as a result of taking NSAIDS, eating highly processed and genetically modified foods, being exposed to pesticides and environmental pollutants, using hand sanitizer, taking antibiotics for the common cold, and other common stressors of modern living. Also keep in mind that our ancestors typically did not live past their fifth or sixth decade of life even though they were eating 100% organic Real Food. If you aren't supplementing, you're depleting. It's as plain and simple as that.

I agree that there are a bunch of dietary supplements that don't work. Many of them don't even contain what's on the label. It's sad, but true. I've carefully vetted the supplements recommended in this book to make sure they're made by reputable companies that implement strict quality control standards, and most importantly, they actually work when used as directed.

It's useful to do some functional medicine lab testing in order to customize a supplement protocol specifically to your unique biochemistry, imbalances, and deficiencies.

However, as a general rule of thumb, there are a few supplements that are useful for most anyone interested in getting the best results on the Autoimmune Protocol. I've listed those supplements here.

Exos Fuel Multivitamin Elite

http://energized.life/product/exos-fuel-multi-vitamin-elite

Most multivitamins contain synthetic vitamins, preservatives, and artificial colors that may actually do more harm than good. Not so with this multi, which contains the most bioavailable forms of necessary B-vitamins, gut-healing vitamin D, anti-inflammatory curcumin, necessary minerals for a healthy thyroid, vitamin K2 to support calcium metabolism, and an evening formula with Relora to reduce stress hormones and prevent late-night food cravings. Visit energized.life and click on products to purchase.

L-Glutamine Powder

http://bit.ly/1K2tx2n

This is the most abundant amino acid in the human body, and your muscles, gastrointestinal tract, and immune system just eats this stuff up during times of real or perceived stress. I recommend taking six scoops of L-Glutamine Powder per day if you're trying to heal yourself from illness or injury, or if you've been under a lot of stress lately.

Proline-Rich Polypeptides Spray

http://energized.life/products

PRPs are made from fresh colostrum and are quite possibly the most important supplement for modulating the immune system in individuals with autoimmune disease. It helps to "heal and seal" the gut, reduce symptoms related to allergies, prevent swelling and tenderness, and improve brain function in Alzheimer's, ADHD, and autism.

Gluten Support Tri-Flora

http://energized.life/products

This probiotic formula contains a synergistic blend of *Saccharomyces boulardii, Lactobacillus,* and *Bifidobacterium.* This combination provides protection against infections and parasites while restoring populations of beneficial microbiota in the gut.

Glutenza

http://energized.life/products

Also referred to as the "gluten pulverizing formula," this blend of digestive enzymes, prebiotics, and probiotics help break down gluten proteins by pulverizing internal and external peptide bonds. It also supports beneficial bacteria in the gut, and is an excellent formula to use during the first 30 days of the Paleo Autoimmune Protocol to help you eliminate any gluten that may still be in your gut.

EPA/DHA Liquid Enhanced

http://bit.ly/1Tuu2qm

These essential fatty acids are crucial for optimal health. DHA is a major component of your brain and eyes, and many experts now recommend 1000 mg of DHA per day to prevent cognitive decline as we age. EPA is a potent anti-inflammatory. Both are required for healing a leaky gut.

How to Reintroduce Foods after Your 30-Day Protocol

I have a feeling you'll get the hang of this Paleo Autoimmune Protocol if you just make a plan to follow the guidelines in this book and also listen to your body. After the initial 30 days, you can start to introduce a wider variety of foods. But please don't do anything crazy! On day 31, it is not in your best interest to stay up all night eating pizza and beer. There's a method to introducing new foods into your dietary protocol, and it doesn't involve throwing every food in your path down the pie hole. Now, let's discuss this method briefly.

Each week after the initial 30 days on the Paleo Autoimmune Protocol, you will try one new category of food. Start with a small amount of the food you are adding and steadily increase that amount as the week progresses. I recommend trying a half cup or one serving of the new food on day 1, one cup or two servings on day 2, and one and a half cups or three servings on day 3 of the week you introduce the new food.

The order in which I recommend adding new food categories after the initial 30 days is as follows:

- — Week 1: Eggs
- — Week 2: Fermented or Raw Dairy
- — Week 3: "Safe" Starches (sweet potatoes, tiger nuts, rice, soaked buckwheat groats)
- — Week 4: Properly Prepared Legumes (soak for 24 hours and cook for 4–8 hours with kelp)
- — Week 5: Chocolate, Coffee, Tea, and Caffeine
- — Week 6: Nightshades (tomatoes, peppers, eggplants)
- — Week 7: Nuts & Seeds
- — Week 8: Red Wine

Notice that except for rice and the pseudograin buckwheat, grains are not added back into the diet even after 90 days. This is not because "the cavemen didn't eat grains" or any other weird ideas the sensationalist media reporters like to say all the silly paleo diet people believe. The real reason behind this recommendation is that this is just what works clinically. Grain consumption has long been associated with an increase in autoimmune disease, gastrointestinal disorders, and even neurological problems. Feel free to add them back into your diet and watch your old symptoms sneak up on you again, but don't say I didn't warn you!

Conclusion

Hopefully after 90 days on the Paleo Autoimmune Protocol, you'll agree that a plate of bacon, eggs, and all-you-can-eat veggies with ghee is a much more satisfying breakfast than a bowl of fat-free cereal or gas-station donuts are any day. People around you will start to notice that your skin looks great, and they'll be wondering what beauty products you've been using. You'll have more energy, a slimmer waistline, and more muscle definition. And if you're ever tempted to throw in the towel and just go back to eating junk food, remember that nothing tastes as good as healthy feels!

Free e-Course

I hope you found this book helpful. To be notified about future books I release, and to get access to my **free** Functional Medicine e-course, go to <u>energized.life</u> and enter your name and email. No gimmicks or spam, I promise! For one-on-one Support, go to <u>energized.life/get-1-on-1-support</u>.

Quick Favor Please?

I'm so grateful that you made the decision to purchase and read this book! If you found it helpful, please take a moment to leave a quick review on Amazon. Your feedback really helps me as an author as well as other readers, and it just takes a moment. Thanks again!

About the Author

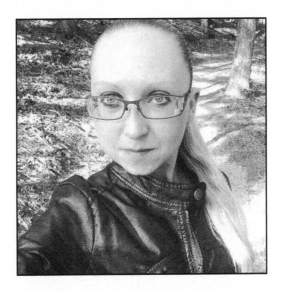

Raised on Frankenberries, Burple, and liquid amoxicillin, Jamie baffled doctors with the worst case of chicken pox ever seen, followed by eczema, asthma, and migraine headaches. The only apparent causes of these health complaints were a pill deficiency and too many bacteria. After calling 1-800-Free-Willy and eventually becoming a member of Greenpeace and PETA, Jamie began to realize that her food choices made an impact on her health as well as the environment. She ditched the "junk" foods and became a vegan, but the nagging health problems just began to escalate. It wasn't until she moved to California in 2003 to study Chinese Medicine that she made the conscious decision to become an omnivore who eats red meat and saturated fat. Within just a few weeks, Jamie began to experience a new level of energy and mental clarity, visible abs, a normal body temperature of 98.6, and no more migraines and asthma attacks. If you'd like to experience a powerful transformation like this, make sure you read all of Jamie's books and sign up for her free Functional Medicine Boot Camp at Energized.Life.

Made in the USA
Charleston, SC
28 December 2016